MENTAL HEALTH STIGMA

How to Overcome Mental Health Stigma in America

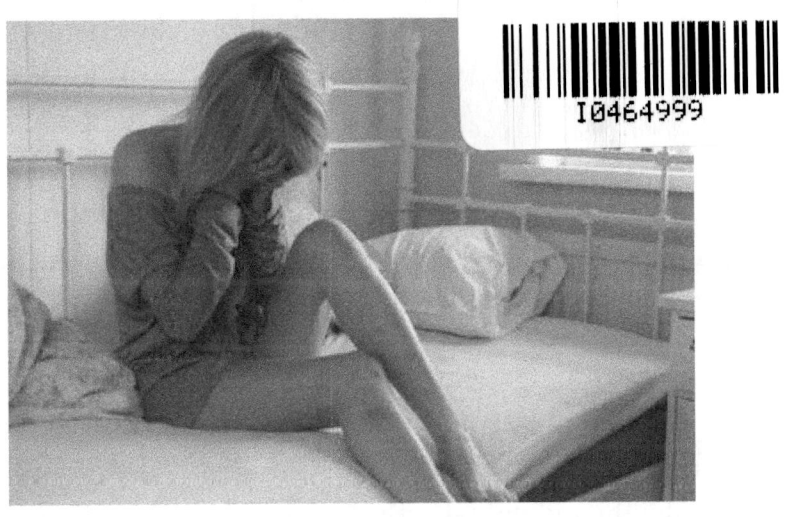

I0464999

By Patricia A Carlisle

Introduction

I want to thank you and congratulate you for choosing the book, *"MENTAL HEALTH STIGMA: How to Overcome Mental Health Stigma in America"*.

This book contains proven steps and strategies on how to overcome mental health stigma in America.

There are a good number of people in the world today that view mental illness side effects as debilitating and uncomfortable, and these disposition most of the time foster stigmas, and discrimination toward individuals with mental health issues. When you admit you have a mental health issue, it can lead to different types of exclusion or discrimination, either inside social circles, or inside of the working environment. This is way most individuals with mental health issues will not seek help for their mental illness.

Mental health stigmas take away from the individual character, and makes negative generalization. Most of the time it is because of the lack of education or false information, tragically; the individual with the mental illness suffers.

Thanks again for choosing this book, I hope you enjoy it!

Patricia A. Carlisle, MSW, CBT

Patricia Carlisle- A Master Social Worker and a Cognitive Behavioral Therapist (CBT) gives out an expression of how important it is for an individual to take into consideration the concept of self-assessment to know what human, technical and conceptual skills they posses to perform or to achieve what they desire, or to deal with everyday life. However, every particular group of people has their own unique set of ideas, traditions and events including the frame of mind according to which people perform but there are many who faces problems and fail to maintain a healthy mind set affecting their behaviors and performance to those around them.

People like Patricia Carlisle are among those who have felt this urge of serving people and helping them out of their mental crisis towards a healthy life. She has experienced some close encounters in her personal life regarding mental health issues in her family and friends that has encouraged her to pursue this as her career.

Currently Patricia Carlisle is serving as a Certified On-Line Cognitive Behavioral Therapist with an extensive 15years of experience using Cognitive Behavior Therapy Techniques. She envisions a world where everyone gets mental health treatment with no mental health stigma and to make it real she has already set up her own Holistic Measure Online Comprehensive Behavioral Healthcare Company after retiring from The Nord Center in The Partial Hospitalization Program (PHP) Dept for 5 years and Murtis H. Taylor Mental Health Center as a mental health counselor, psychological support technician and case manager for 10 years to emulsify her skills more professionally. Along with this, she has wrote down her passion as a clinician in 25 or more short books to help individuals and families get their life back, freeing them of the restraints of negative thinking, anxiety and depression by using different approaches. She is highly appreciated among her clients for her flexibility and professionalism of dealing with them graciously.

To reach her, make use of her direct website address: http://therapist2013.wix.com/e-therapy . As she is ready to inspire hope and contribute to health and well-being by providing the best online health care through comprehensive practice, education and research.

TABLE OF CONTENT

Chapter 1

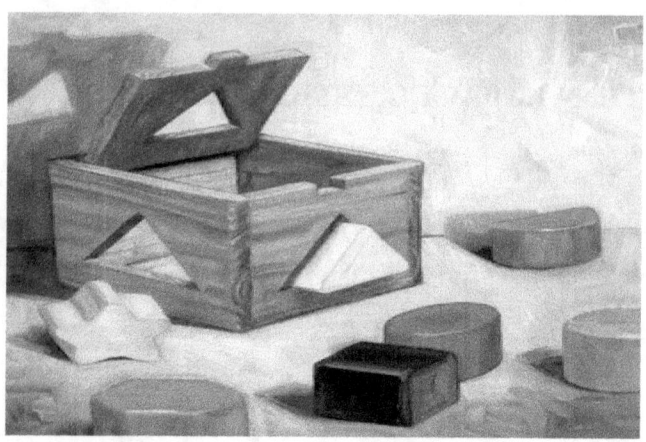

DISCRIMINATION IMPACT OF STIGMAS

Stigma can prompt discrimination. Discrimination may be obvious and immediate, for example, someone making a negative comment about your mental illness or your treatment. On the other hand, it might be unexpected or modest, for example, by keeping away from you because they expect you to be unsteady, savage, or dangerous because of your mental health condition. You may start to judge yourself.

The destructive impact of stigma can include:

- Reluctance to look for help or treatment.

- Stop seeing family, friends, colleagues, or others you know.

- Fewer doors open for employment, school, and social settings.

- Bullying, physical roughness, or aggravation from others.

- Health insurance that doesn't cover your mental health treatment.

- The conviction that you'll never have the capacity to succeed at a specific tasks, or that you can't improve your circumstances.

Chapter 2

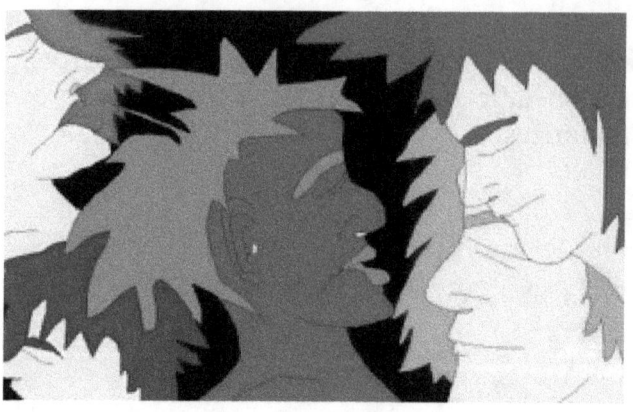

HOW TO MANAGE STIGMA IN AMERICA

Here are a few ways you can manage stigma:

- **Get treatment.** You may be hesitant to maintain your require treatment. Try not to let the fear of being marked with a mental illness keep you from looking for help. Treatment can help you understand your illness, as well as finding out the cause, and help diminish symptoms that interfere with your work and life.

- **Don't let stigma give you self-uncertainty and disgrace.** Stigma doesn't simply originate from others it can come for you. You might accept that your condition is an indication of your shortcoming, or you should have the capacity to control it without help. Look for mental guidance, educate yourself about your condition, and unite with others with mental illness to help you increase self-interest, and overcome harmful self-judgment.

- **Don't separate yourself.** If you have a mental illness, don't hesitant to educate people concerning it. Your family, companions, ministry, or individuals from your group can offer you support. Connect with individuals you trust for the sympathy, support and understanding you need.

- **Don't see yourself as your mental illness.** You are not your illness. So instead of saying "I'm bipolar, "say "I have bipolar". Instead of calling yourself "a schizophrenic," say "I have schizophrenia."

- **Join a support group.** Some neighborhood and national gatherings, for example, the National Alliance of Mental Illness (NAMI), offer nearby projects, and internet resources that help decrease stigma by teaching individuals with mental illness, their families, and the overall population. Also, states and government have offers and projects, for example, those who attention is on professional restoration, or the Department of Veterans Affairs (VA), offer support for individuals with mental health issues.

- **Get help at school.** If you or your child has a mental illness that effect learning, find out what plans and projects may offer assistance. Discrimination against students due to a mental health condition is illegal, and instructors and schools are obliged to accommodate students. Talk with educators, teachers, or managers about the best approach and resources.

- **Speak out against stigma.** Consider discussing stigma in letters to the editorial manager or on the internet. It can help ingrain courage in others, also challenge a relative about mental health, and teach the general population about mental illness.

Figuring out how to admit you have an illness, and decide what you need to do to treat it, such as finding support, and helping educate others can have a major effect.

Despite the fact an expected 44 million adults and 13.7 million children in America have a diagnosable mental illness every year, the issue of mental health stays encompassed by stigma and misconception. However, the issue of mental illness requires more prominent consideration as an important 21st century general health challenge. Among the large number of Americans, less than half get help, despite the fact that 80 to 90 percent of mental illness is treatable with prescriptions, and different treatment choices.

Mental illness takes a huge toll on people, families, and society. Despite the critical effect, mental illness is a huge financial expense. Treatment for symptoms alone is calculated to cost $83 billion yearly. Stigma is overpowering because many consider mental illness as part of a person's character opposed to a genuine illness, similar to other illnesses, such as diabetes.

Treatment for mental illness as a genuine 21st century general health test means:

- Concentrating on particular age, racial/ethnic, and sexual orientation related danger elements.

- Enhancing state funded education to reduce stigma so that more individuals are eager, and ready to look for help.

- Training the specialists in screening for mental illness, and referring patients to mental health services they require.

Chapter 3

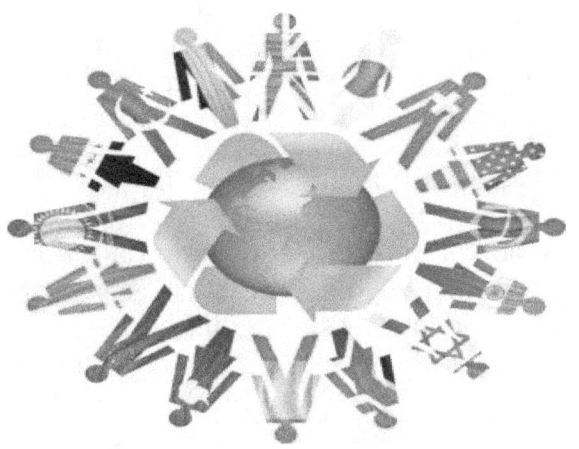

MENTAL ILLNESS STATISTICS

Mental illness can add other problems such as, dietary problems including anorexia and bulimia, addictive issue, alcohol abuse, identity issue, and others.

In a National Institute of Health (NIH) review, stated America adults led in 2008, age, sex and race variables were broke down among the individuals who had genuine mental illness. Females were more influenced than males, more youthful Americans more than more seasoned Americans, with differing results across ethnicity. Understanding the effect of sexual orientation, age and ethnic/racial contrasts is critical in outlining projects to decrease the pervasiveness of mental illness, and in focusing on powerful mediations.

Depression and Post-traumatic stress disorder (PTSD), are found more in ladies while different issue, similar to alcohol abuse and withdraw identity issue, are found more in men. The basics for these sexual orientation contrasts are to some extent connected to natural components, such as hormones.

There are additionally other dangerous elements that excessively influence ladies with mental illness, including roughness, low financial status, salary disparity, secondary status in society, and anxiety which can develop at work, and children care obligations. Given these circumstances, ladies are more inclined to experience the ill effects of a particular mental illness, for example, depression and anxiety, additionally 50 percent more women is reluctant to utilize mental health services than men.

In addition, children and young adults are at high risk for developing mental illness, with 13 percent of youth in the United States, 18 years old youth will meet the criteria for one of the most predominant mental diseases; such as anxiety issues, anger issues, dietary issues, discouragement, hyperactivity issue, and behavioral issue. Although there is some debate about whether issues like ADHD and dipolar issue are over-analyzed in American kids, youth are undeniable in danger for mental health issues that can be made worse by environmental components, for example, manhandle and ignored, a distressing learning environment and media impacts that produce a perfect body type.

Chapter 4

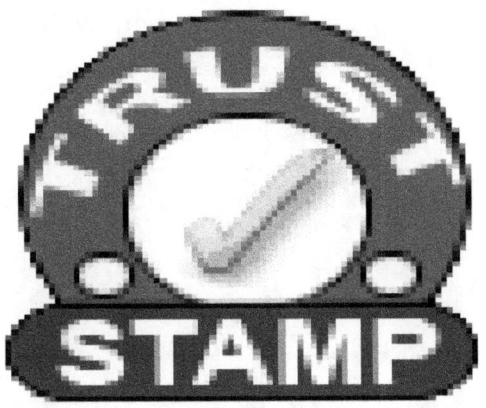

HOW TO STAMP OUT STIGMA

Understanding the elements that add to mental illness is the first step to stamping out stigma. Another step to reducing stigma is education; you can help the general public understand how some mental illnesses may have an organic and neurological base, and is not a character imperfection or the individual's fault. Another step is expanding your effort to educate others by talking to family. General mental health training will help you to recognize symptoms of mental illness in yourself, friends and family, and will give you the information you need to help you choose the right support program.

You can become frustrated by the way mental health specialists neglect to identify mental illness when you go to them for help. Medical Doctors are not prepared to be mental health providers. 50% of the individuals who meet the criteria for mental illness are found by their medical doctor. A late study found that doctors neglect to identify around 66% of their patients who come to them with mental health problems.

Also, mental health specialists are frequently unable to distinguish the symptom for mental illness. Doctors and therapists must be able to identify early symptoms of mental illness, and have the ability to address patients that need help from a qualified mental health experts. By recognizing mental illness early, mental health experts can possibly change the way you feel, and eliminate the impacts of feeling awful while experiencing different symptoms of illness.

Chapter 5

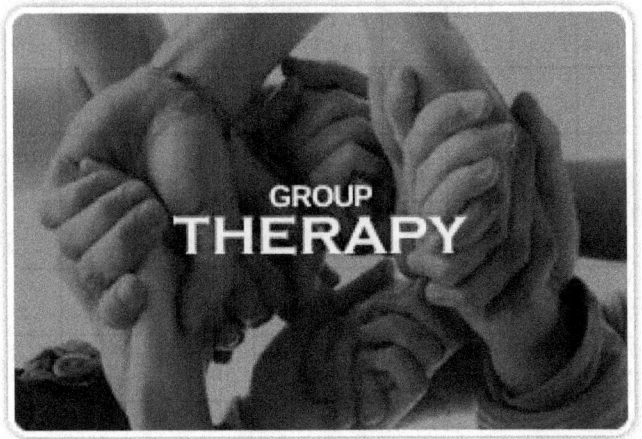

TREATMENT FOR MENTAL ILLNESS

Treatment for mental illness can consist of, psychotherapy, solutions, social support, and life style changes. Support from family, friends and groups are fundamental in mental health treatment. Also, behavioral medications, physical fitness, better nutrition, and rest can lower anxiety, this will add to your general health and empower you to deal with your mental illness.

Mental Health Month is a good time to bring mental health issues to light. Focus on the public, diminishing the stigma surrounding mental issue. Coordinate mental health into thought and treatment systems that will allow advance discovery and treatment for mental illness in the future.

Absence of Information

More adults and their families should get educated about the causes, and the effect of mental illness among people. They should understand mental illness is not "typical" to the growing process, and recovery is possible. Having no knowledge or understanding about health centers leaves many without answers for their illness.

Absence of Competent Health Care Professionals

Health care experts, such as, specialist, mental health therapist, doctor's aides, and others, can stop stigma on adults with mental illness. Sometimes experts may decline to consider these sicknesses important, reject their patients, or give misdiagnoses.

Absence of Understanding

Associations may be ignorant of the signs and effect of mental illness among adults. Regardless of the fact that the illness is apparent, those in an organization, a working environment, or a religious association may accept the issues as "reasonable", or "ordinary", or adversely judge that individual in view of the illness.

Chapter 6

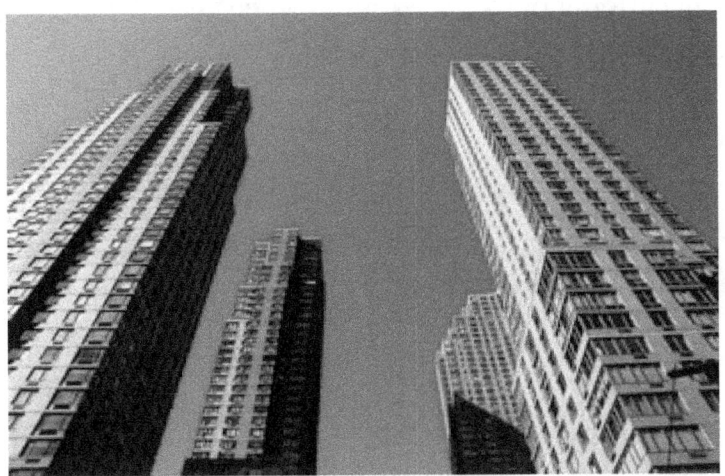

REFINING CORPORATION MEETINGS

In spite of the fact the message of mental illness must be further refined in business to reduce stigma, some corporations are incorporating topics such as:

- Treatment meets expectations. More adults with mental illness can enhance and recover.

- More adults with mental illness must attempt to meet difficulties with courage to overcome apprehension, segregation, and absence of resources.

- Helping other people helps you (the Helper's Principle). If you are an adult with a mental illness, you help yourself when you help other people. If you are in a position to help an individual with a mental illness, doing so will support your self-interest, and feeling of self-esteem.

- It is essential for an adult to reside at home with no fear of feeling wrong.

- There is promise for development, and recovery, for feeling better about you. "Would you be able to improve?" Yes.

Chapter 7

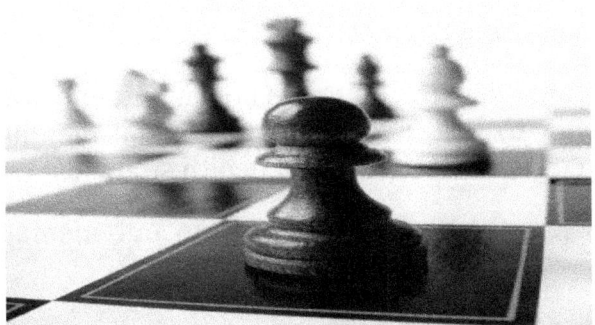

GENERAL STRATEGIES

One strategy to help stop stigma is to help others understand adults with mental illness by having group meetings, talking to a mental health specialists and volunteers, such as, home health care helpers, meals-on-wheels volunteers, and health care providers, all of the above must be educated about mental illness.

Community groups have a great chance to reach more adults through their get-togethers and group supervision. One thought in particular was a "Senior Mental Health Corporation" for adults, made up of both clients and additional people, who discuss the meaning of mental health, and talk about medications and side-effects. Corporation should present more projects on mental health issues in groups as well as support adult clients with mental illness, and advocate at State and national levels. Other ways to advocate is through associate advising, and tutoring projects. This is an important process to reach more people about mental illness.

Conclusion

Thank you again for choosing this book!

I hope this book was able to help you to see how mental health stigma have a tendency to hold negative beliefs about mental illness, and what you can do to stop mental health stigma.

The next step is to practice the steps to stamp out mental health stigma.

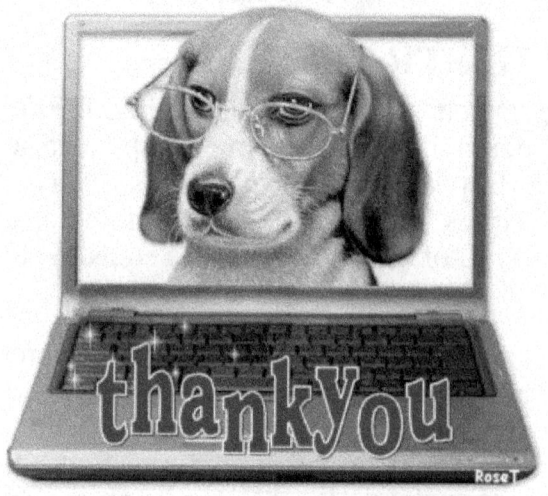

Finally, if you enjoyed this book would you be kind enough to leave a review for this book on Amazon? It'd be greatly appreciated!

Thank you and good luck!

Preview Of 'MOOD SWINGS: How to control your mood swings to avoid emotional rollercoaster's'

Chapter 1
MOOD SWINGS

A mood swing is just a recognizable change in one's mood or enthusiastic state. Everyone has mood swings and they are a characteristic piece of a lot of people's lives. We get happy, we get sad, We have a time of feeling like we are on top of the world and in charge, and sometimes, we feel drained, dormant and whipped. Little mood swings are a piece of the vast majority's lives.

On the other hand, a few individuals' mood swings are so drastic, fast or genuine; that they meddle with that singular's working in ordinary life. Bipolar issue is the best sample of an issue that is described by mood swings-from hyper to discourage. You can, notwithstanding, have mood swings between any two moods or feelings, pitiful to furious, cheerful to pensive. Let us identify some of the reasons for mood swings in individuals.

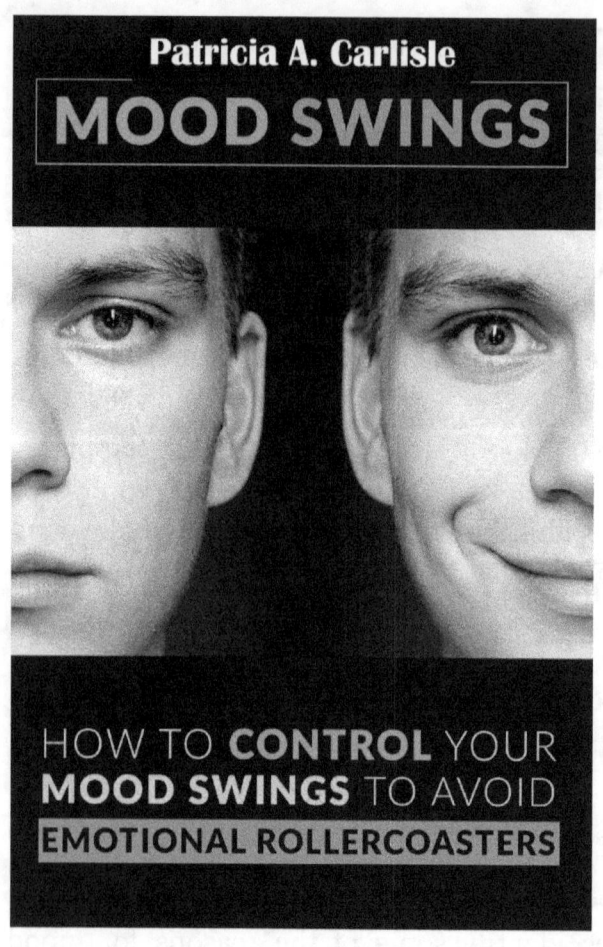

Patricia A. Carlisle

MOOD SWINGS

HOW TO **CONTROL** YOUR
MOOD SWINGS TO AVOID
EMOTIONAL ROLLERCOASTERS

check out the rest of (MOOD SWINGS: How to control your mood swings to avoid emotional rollercoaster's) on Amazon.com

Check Out My Other Books

Below you'll find some of my other popular books that are popular on Amazon and Kindle as well. Alternatively, you can visit my author page on Amazon to see other work done by me.

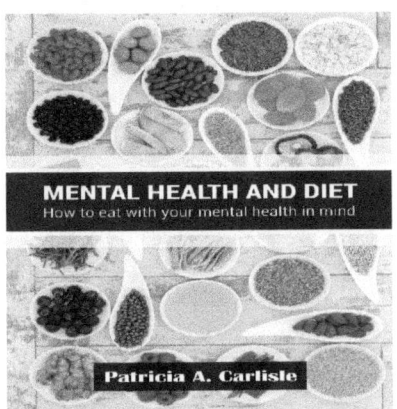

Mental Health and diet: How to eat with your mental health in mind

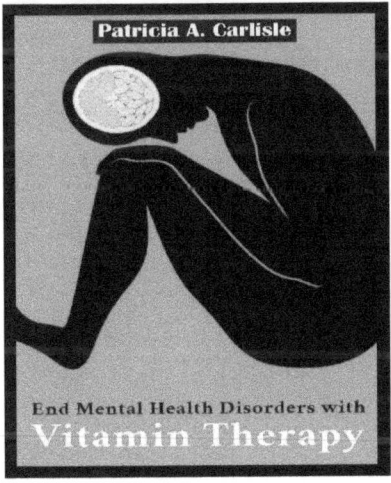

End Mental Disorders with vitamin therapy.

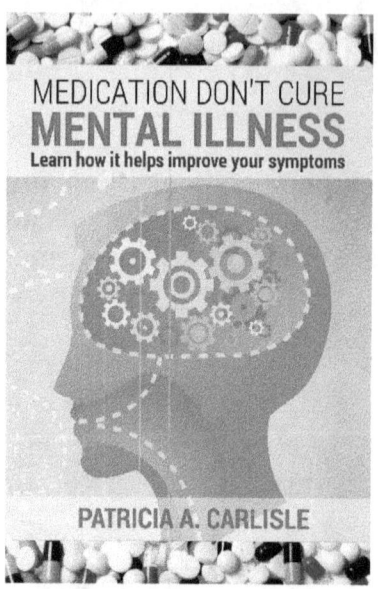

MEDICATION DON'T CURE MENTAL ILLNESS: Learn how it helps improve your symptoms.

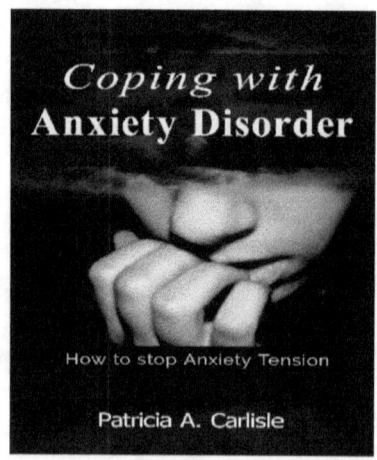

Coping with Anxiety Disorder: How to stop Anxiety Tension.

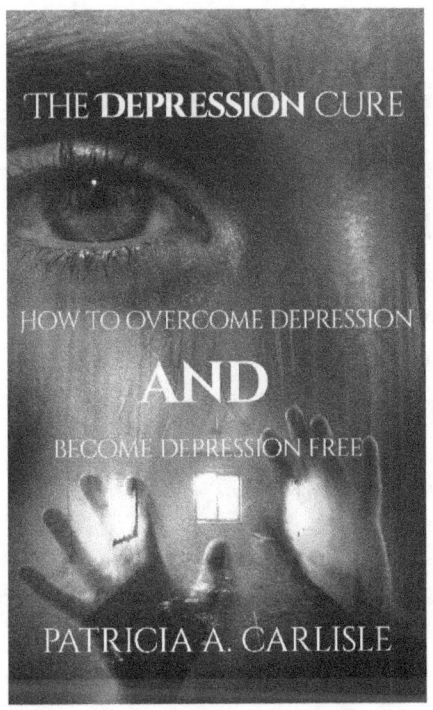

THE DEPRESSION CURE: How to overcome depression and become depression free.

BONUS: SUBSCRIBE TO THE FREE BOOK

Beginners Guide to Yoga & Meditation

"Stressed out? Do You Feel Like The World Is Crashing Down Around You? Want To Take A Vacation That Will Relax Your Mind, Body And Spirit? Well this Easy To Read Step By Step

E-Book Makes It All Possible!"

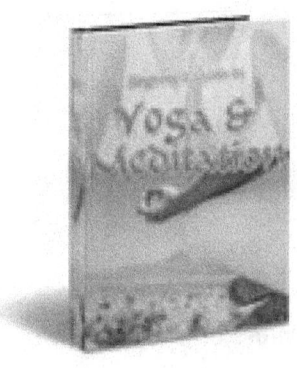

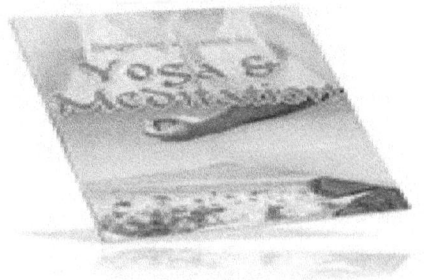

Instructions on how to join our mailing list, and receive a free copy of "Yoga and Meditation" can be found in any of my Kindle eBooks.

NOTES

NOTES

NOTES

NOTES

NOTES

NOTES

NOTES